Aromatherapy Recipes for Beginners

100 DIY Essential Oil Recipes for House Cleaning, Personal Beauty, and Optimal Health

Ellie Jones

© 2016

Disclaimer

Table of Contents

Introduction

Aromatherapy is defined as the use of plant materials and oils, such as aromatic compounds and essential oils, in order to beneficially alter a person's physical and emotional well being. Aromatherapy has been used as a time of complementary therapy just as much as it has been long offered as a time of alternative medicine.

People who specialize in aromatherapy are known as aromatherapists, and blend a number of different essential oils to be applied trough inhalation, massage, and

The use of essential oils is the heart of aromatherapy. Some kinds of essential oils, such as tea tree for example, have been shown to have some positive effects for mental and physical health, such as fighting against viral and bacterial infections. This use of essential oils has been used for hundreds of years, all the way back in the ancient civilizations of the Egyptians, Indians, Chinese, and Greeks and Romans who used the oils as perfumes and cosmetics. However, the concept of using essential oil in this manner did not develop into true aromatherapy until European scientists explored the topic in greater depth in the 1900s. It was during this time that the benefits of essential oils began to be truly explored beyond their simple perfume and cosmetic functions and to aid in benefiting physical and emotional health.

The health uses of aromatherapy were put to the test in World War II, where they were used as an anti-septic in treating wounded soldiers on both sides of the conflict.

In essence, aromatherapy explores both technical and creative knowledge. It explores creative knowledge in that researchers can envision new essential oil scents and combinations by knowing the characteristics of them. The technical knowledge comes from knowing about the chemicals within the oils and how they can help the human body.

How Do Essential Oils Help the Body?

The primary part of the body that essential oils affect the most is the mind, especially the component of the brain that controls one's emotion. Think of the molecules within essential oils as the key that unlocks the nerve receptors in your nostril. This aroma impression is immediately sent to your limbic system, which is where all of your memories are stored and you perceive the resulting emotions out of those memories. When the limbic system has been stimulated in this manner, it releases chemicals that directly affect your nervous system such as serotonin, which reduces pain and anxiety levels.

This is why inhaling or coming into contact with essential oils can give you a very pleasurable emotional feeling. At the very least, essential oils will be able to give you emotional balance.

The best way to give you immediate relief in this manner with essential oils is to inhale or diffuse the oils directly. Using chamomile as an example, simply place two or three drops onto a handkerchief and then breathe it in under your nose deeply. Alternatively, you can allow the chamomile (or any essential oil for that matter) to diffuse into the air with the aid of an aromatherapy lamp that consists of a basin to hold a mixture of essential oils and water to diffuse the resulting scent. A candle warms the basin from underneath it.

Peppermint, chamomile, lemon, and basil are the most common essential oils that are diffused into the air in this manner.

Essential oils can also heal the actual body rather than just the mind. For instance, it's easy for the oils to be absorbed through the body's skin and find their way into the individual cells to cleanse, tone, or balance them. This adds an entirely new dimension to the healing effects that other healing practices, such as massages, compresses, and baths can bring. Essential oils are concentrated, so they can compose at least three percent of the blends that are used in these other healing products and practices. The possibilities are endless, and will consist of a large number of the recipes that we will explore in this book. Essential oils can be added to bath water to benefit the skin, for instance, and there are so many different recipes and combinations to do so, each with their own benefits.

Last but not least, essential oils will work wonders on you beyond your mind and body by benefiting your spirit. While prayer and/or meditation is perhaps the best thing that can give your spirit a boost, the effects of essential oils are a close second and go hand in hand with both your mind and body.

It's perfectly understandable if you are still doubtful of the benefits that aromatherapy can bring you. However, you shouldn't be too quick to draw any conclusions either. Aromatherapy is most commonly known as a technique for relaxation, but it can just as easily if not more effectively be used to treat a variety of different healthy issues. If you've been looking for a new way to relax and boost your health, aromatherapy just might be it. Besides, it's very hard to resist the excellent smells that most of the essential oils in our one hundred and one recipes produce.

Next, let's go over what the specific benefits of aromatherapy are, primarily the health related ones. The first is that aromatherapy reduces stress. Doesn't the very word 'aromatherapy' sound so relaxing on its own? There's real science that backs up that aromatherapy is beneficial to stress. Several studies have shown that patients who use aromatherapy feel significantly less pain and stress in stressful situations, especially when compared to patients who were not using aromatherapy. In fact, stress relief is actually easily one of the most widespread uses of aromatherapy in general. The compounds that are featured in many of the various essential oils are classified as relaxants and naturally soothe the body. These mixtures are also very simple and well studied in order to back up the idea that they work. Some of the best specific essential oils for dealing with stress are peppermint, lavender, lemon oil, and bergamot. Of these, lemon oil is believed to be the most effective.

Aromatherapy is also very effective at managing depression. The vibrant and citrus based aromas and essential oils in particular can reduce depression and put a smile in your face. This one is arguably more important than stress because most of the pharmaceutical anti-depressants on the market, no matter how effective they may be at reducing depression, still come with a long list of unwanted side effects. While we're not suggesting that aromatherapy should fully take the place of anti-depressants or other anti-depression measures in your treatment (if depression is an issue you're going through), we are saying that it can be an addition to whatever treatment you are using currently. The best specific essential oils for managing depression are lavender, chamomile, peppermint, and jasmine.

Managing stress and depression is one thing, but managing physical pain is something else entirely. Nonetheless, aromatherapy has still very pain management properties. So the real question becomes if aromatherapy can relieve physical pain, then why would you not try to take advantage of it? Lavender, clary sage, juniper, chamomile, rosemary, eucalyptus, and peppermint have all been used by professional athletes even for pain relief, and they can just as easily be applied in your personal home life.

Stress, depression, and physical pain are easily the top three most widespread uses for aromatherapy in dealing with physical pain. But there are still many more health benefits that are worth a little discussion:

- Low blood pressure levels. Aromatherapy has been shown to reduce blood pressure levels in patients who have hypertension. The reason or this is because many essential oils contain very relaxing properties that allow you to relax and bring your blood pressure levels down to a very healthy level.

- Improved memory. Among older people, suffering from memory loss is easily one of the most frightening diseases to fear. Unfortunately, it's also a disease that has been steadily increasing among older people as well, especially the ability to keep short term memories. Memory loss diseases, such as Alzheimer's, are still relatively incurable even in today's day and age. Nonetheless, that doesn't mean that the onset of memory loss diseases can be slowed down or the effects of them decreased. Aromatherapy has been used as a type of supplemental treatment to detention and similar diseases in the past and present. But it doesn't just end with older people. Research has revealed that even younger patients can boost their memory capacity for a temporary amount of time after aromatherapy treatment. This boost to your brain will definitely aid you in all walks of life.

- More energy. We require energy just to pull ourselves through the normal stresses of life. Energy pills and coffee are two of the most common things we use to give ourselves the extra boost of energy we need. However, even coffee and energy bars can hurt your body if you take too much of them. This is where aromatherapy comes in to provide you with an alternative way to get this energy boost. A lot of the essential oils that aromatherapy makes use of are able to raise energy levels by increasing blood flow and circulation, which helps to stimulate both your mind and body, but without the side effects that other substances and medications can give you. The best essential oils for boosting your energy include rosemary, sage, jasmine, tea tree, cinnamon, and clove.

- Improved Recovery Times. After being physically injured or fatigued, many of us turn to pharmaceuticals that can shorten our recovery times and get us back on track faster. However, many different kinds of essential oils can do this exact same thing. The reason for this is because they provide extra oxygen to the blood and increase the actual rate of the blood flow. This makes the internal healing process much faster for everything from an internal illness to an external wound. Plus, many essential oils contain anti-microbial properties that provide reinforced protection to the body as well. All in all, essential oils contain the properties necessary to reduce the severity of wounds, shorten the time that discomfort is felt, and accelerate the overall healing process as a whole.

- Improved Headaches. We all get headaches at various times, and the worst headaches can be enough to put us out of action for one day. But just like how we rely too often on pharmaceuticals to speed up recovery times, we also rely on the same medications to get us through the worst of the headaches as well. However, essential oils and aromatherapy in particular is among the most powerful solutions for not only getting rid of your current bad headache, but for reducing the chances of developing another one in the future as well. Some of the specific essential oils that have been known to reduce the effects of headaches include sandalwood, rosemary, eucalyptus, and peppermint. These oils can be mixed together and then applied to the temples, neck, and scalp in order to gain the fastest relief.

- Better Sleep at Night. The average adult needs at least eight hours of sleep each night in order to stay optimally healthy, but unfortunately, the average adult only gets around five to six hours of that sleep. The result is feeling fatigued, a loss of energy, and unproductive days. Aromatherapy is easily one of the best solutions available for getting back into a natural sleep schedule and is feeling energized for the next day. The best essential oils that have these sedative effects include rose, chamomile, lavender, jasmine, and sandalwood.

- A Boosted Immune System. The immune system is the system in your body that prevents you from getting sick. If the human body lacked an immune system, each and every one of us would be getting sick from bacteria and infections all of the time, and average human life expectancy would be drastically reduced. Some people have a weakened immune system and the results are devastating in both their personal and professional lives. Fortunately, the essential oils in aromatherapy contain strong anti-bacterial effects that protect you from these infections and bacteria, such as oregano, lemon, cinnamon, eucalyptus, and peppermint.

- Improved Digestion. The effects of aromatherapy on the digestive system are arguably the least researched topic of aromatherapy in general. Nonetheless, the limited amount of research that has been conducted on the topic of the relation between aromatherapy and digestion has strongly suggested that there is a very positive relationship. It is believed that essential oils such as fennel, ginger, sage, and lavender can increase food metabolism, reduce bloating and constipation, and speed up the overall digestive process.

How to Use Aromatherapy

There are three primary ways that you can use aromatherapy, and the overwhelming majority of the one hundred and one recipes that we will talk about will fall under one or more of the three methods.

The first method is by massage or at least by direct contact with the skin. Essential oils have high concentration levels, and are often mixed in with carrier oils such as almond, grape seed, or olive. Carrier oils are needed in order to spread the essential oils as much as possible and to prevent a negative reaction with the skin. In aromatherapy, this allows the essential oils to be better rubbed and soaked in by the skin.

The second method is by breathing in the oils through your nostrils, and within this one method, there are quite a few more methods that are used to inhale essential oils. One such 'sub-method' is to drop the oils into a handkerchief or cloth and then breathe them in when holding them under your nose. Another such 'sub-method' is to drop the oils into a bowl of hot water and then inhaling the resulting steam. A third and final 'sub-method' is to get the vapor of the oils to fill the entire room by using an essential oil burner that is designed specifically for the task.

The third and final method for applying aromatherapy combines the first two methods. Add a few drops of essential oils to a warm bath, and then breathe in the resulting vapors while the oils soak your skin. This is the most relaxing way to use aromatherapy.

Finally, the essential oils of aromatherapy can also be applied into a number of different home cleaning services. The cleaner your home is, the healthier you will be.

The point of this introduction has been to teach you that there are two primary functions for why you would want to consider using aromatherapy: 1. it's incredibly relaxing, and 2. it comes with a number of important health benefits that you would expect from more traditional medications regardless of whether you apply it directly to your body or use it to clean your home.

Just a handful of the health benefits we have told you about from aromatherapy is the ability to speed up healing processes, to let you sleep better, to reduce the onset of headaches, to boost energy levels, to calm down stress and depression, increase blood circulation, boost your immune system, and speed up the digestive process.

Taken as a whole, aromatherapy is a very fascinating subject that serves as a viable alternative to traditional medicine. The heart and soul of aromatherapy is the use of essential oils that are applied in the three methods (and sub-methods) that we told you about. While most doctors wouldn't recommend that you use aromatherapy to supplement any medications or medical treatments you are currently using, there is no harm done in using aromatherapy as an addition to them.

Aromatherapy has existed in some shape or form for several thousand years, and ever since the 11th Century, numerous cultures have properly removed essential oils from their source plant materials and utilized them for a number of different functions. The four countries that have made the most effective and widespread use of aromatherapy would have to be France, England, India, and the United States. If you've been cautious about aromatherapy even up until this point, just know it's a therapy that's been used by millions of people around the globe for thousands of years.

The last topic of aromatherapy that we will talk about before moving onto our one hundred and one recipes is synergy. Synergy is defined as the combination of essential oils into creating a more powerful effect than each of the oils would have had by themselves. Synergy is going to be the heart of each of the recipes that we will go into, because our recipes do exactly that: most of them combine two or more essential oils in order to create a more soothing, relaxing, and health beneficial effect.

Last but not least, don't forget to consult with a professional aromatherapist if necessary. The reason we recommend this is because some essential oils can cause allergic reactions, and the best person to help discover which oils are causing a potential allergic reaction in you (if any are at all) would be an aromatherapist. Additionally, mixing together two or more essential oils together can make them toxic and/or negative side-effect inducing if you use the wrong ones. Again, a professional aromatherapist will ensure that you don't make this kind of mistake.

There are a nearly infinite number of different essential oil combinations, and one hundred and one recipes can only cover a small percentage of those combinations. The ones that we have included in this book are the most popular and effective ones, and are also the easiest to apply.

100 Aromatherapy Recipes

1 – Purifying Tea Tree Peppermint Travel Mist

We're going to start out with one of the most refreshing recipes in this entire book. Regardless of whether you are taking a long road trip or are just driving on your way to work, this recipe will still provide you with the full power benefits of tea tree and the freshness that peppermint provides.

For ingredients, take one teaspoon of grain alcohol, fifteen drops of tea tree essential oil, ten drops of peppermint essential oil, four ounces of clean water, and fifteen drops of tangerine essential oil.

Place the grain alcohol into a spray bottle, and then add each of the essential oils before shaking to mix thoroughly. Then, add the water and shake vigorously again. You can then remove the cap and mist the air that is around you. Remember to avoid getting any of the mist into any sensitive areas such as your eyes or ears.

2 – Aura Cacia Essential Oil Blend

This is a completely natural solution that can be used for everything from car cleaning to energizing yourself, leaving behind a minty and yet citrusy smelling clean aroma.

Combine over twenty ounces of clean water with eight ounces of white vinegar, at least on tablespoon of liquid castile soap, and fifty drops of the pep talk essential solutions blend. Proceed to place all of these ingredients into a spray bottle, and then spray the mixture into a paper towel or a clean cloth and proceed to wipe whatever surfaces you need cleaned clean.

3 – Car Carpet Cleaning Powder

This is a very natural and simple recipe to make. Powder should always be your number one choice when you clean the carpets in your car, especially powder recipes that contain corn starch and/or baking soda. Both of these products can better absorb the odors in your vehicle and eliminate the actual signs of grime and grease.

The ingredients for this article are a one half cup of baking soda, another half cup of corn starch, fifty drops of the first response essential solutions blend, and then a half teaspoon of castile soap flakes.

Your goal in mixing these products together is to create the powder like we talked about. The resulting powder should be slightly damp, but still able to be sprinkled nicely over your car carpet. Then, use a brush to get the powder into the stains of the carpet. Give the powder a minimum of twelve hours to sit before vacuuming it up. Your car carpets should be as good as new!

4 – Carpet Deodorizing Powder

There are very few places in your home that can collect as much dust, dirt, and grime as the carpets. However, simply vacuuming your carpets can only do so much. It can remove most of the visible dust and dirt, but it can never truly freshen your carpets to make them truly healthy you to breathe in. This is where the carpet deodorizing powder recipe steps in.

The ingredients to this powerful recipe are incredibly simple: one teaspoon of bergamot (a type of essential oil), mixed with one cup of baking soda.

Mix the two thoroughly together into a bowl. The result should be a very damp powder similar in texture to the last recipe. Store this resulting recipe in a container and sprinkle when needed over a messy area of the carpets. After the powder has sat on the carpet for at least fifteen minutes, proceed to vacuum over it as usual. There are few recipes that will be as purifying for your carpets as this one.

5 – Winter Blend

This is a recipe that you will absolutely not want to directly ingest! Take five drops of bay essential oil and mix it in with five more drops each of fennel seed essential oil and anise essential oil.

Next, blend the two together in a glass bowl or cup. Then, place the mixture into a diffuser and breathe in deeply. Just be sure that the mixture does not come into contact with your skin or be swallowed through your mouth. When you have finished with the blend, you can then set it aside (make sure it is out of children). The essential oils will continue to work together, and the resulting aroma that you smell in your home will be very refreshing and help to restore true peace of mind.

6 – Patio Outdoor Spray

This is a recipe that will make you want to stay outside on your patio for as long and as often as possible, so long as you enjoy the delightful smell of lemon.

For ingredients, gather two ounces worth of clean water, twenty drops of lemon tree essential oil, dozen drops each of citronella essential oil, lemon eucalyptus essential oil, and vetiver essential oil each, followed by five drops of cedar wood essential oil. Combine the ingredients in a bottle, and then shake and spray outdoors and enjoy the smell.

7 – Briquette

This recipe is designed to get rid of the odor you smell from your garbage disposal with a very clean and citrus scent from lemon tea tree essential oil. This is a good mixture to have on hand either in the garage or underneath the sink every day.

For ingredients, you'll need a fresh lemon a cup of salt and baking soda each, and then two tablespoons of lemon tea tree essential oil.

Start by cutting the lemon into four equal sizes, and then pulp them together in an appropriate food processor as you see fit. Proceed to add the lemons to the salt and baking soda mix, and then stir them together until they are well blended and turn out in the form of a paste. Add the lemon tea tree essential oil and continue to mix it together.

Pour the mixtures into a baking mold tray (preferably one made out of silicone), and then allow one to two days for the mixtures to dry. Once they have, you can then pop them out of the mold tray and store in a glass jar or container.

When using, simply run one of the pieces through a dispenser with hot, clean water.

8 – Summertime Bergamot and Lavender Room Spray

The definition of a perfect, aroma-filed summers day is this recipe right here. This recipe combines bergamot essential oil with lavender to create the perfect summertime aroma.

The ingredients are eight drops each of the bergamot and lavender essential oils, mixed with four ounces of clean water.

This combination will need to be mixed into a spray bottle. Shake the bottle very well before each use and then mist the room with the liquid. In order to get the most benefits out of his mixture, feel free to spray more out of the bottle than you'll think you need. The result is very refreshing and energizing.

9 – Grapefruit Tile Scrub

Housecleaning is always a pain, but aromatherapy can help freshen up each experience thanks to the countless recipes available that take care of and disinfect your home and give your nostrils the purifying aroma they need at the same time. This recipe is no exception.

Combine two tablespoons of baking soda with another two tablespoons of sea salt, and then take three drops of tea tree essential oil and peppermint essential oil, and then fifteen drops of grapefruit essential oil

Mix the ingredients together while keeping them fully dry. You can then sprinkle the resulting product over tile in the kitchen or the tub with the bathroom. Use hot water and a clean sponge or cloth to scrub and rinse to complete the process.

10 – Spray Cleaner

This is a recipe that serves multiple functions. It's also a very simple recipe that is composed of just four ingredients: two teaspoons of lavender essential oil, two cups of warm and clean water, and then a one half teaspoon each of sodium borate and liquid soap (preferably unscented).

The process to mixing these recipes together, however, is a little more complicated. Start by dissolving the sodium borate into the water in a spray bottle, and then add the lavender and liquid soap. Stir accordingly as you see fit. Shake the bottle vigorously before use and then spray onto the surface, and proceed to wipe it clean with a cloth.

This is a general purpose spray cleaner that can be used to clean up a number of different messes in your home, while simultaneously providing you with the fragrant benefits of aroma therapy.

11 – Lemon Oil Oven Cleaner

With this cleaner we're going to get a little more specific instead of general purpose. Mot oven cleaners on the market can yield a number of harsh fumes, but that will be replaced with the more fresh aroma delivered by the lemon essential oil.

For ingredients, you'll need a one quarter cup of vinegar, one and a half cups of baking soda, a half cup of liquid soap (preferably one that is unscented), and then two teaspoons of lemon tea tree essential oil.

Mix all of these ingredients thoroughly together in a bowl until a paste begins to form. Use a brush to essentially paint the inside of your oven, but try to avoid the heating elements of the inside. Once you have painted the inside, shut the door and leave your oven alone for a full day. This means avoid re-opening the oven door or turning the oven on.

After a day has passed, soak a sponge in some warm water and then re-wipe over the entire inside of your oven. The result will be a very clean oven, as well some very purifying aroma being sent into your nostrils.

12 – Room and Body Mist

This is a recipe that combines germanium with lavender essential oils to provide both your room and body with a mist that's extremely soothing.

Take a dozen drops each of lavender and geranium essential oils, and then mix them in with warm, clean water in a spray bottle. Shake the bottle very well until the combination has been mixed very thoroughly.

You can either spray the mist into a room to help freshen the air, or you can apply it directly to your skin (be sure to avoid any sensitive areas, including the eyes and ear lobes). Always give the bottle a little shake before use.

13 – Toned Down Travel Mist

This recipe is a toned down version of our first recipe in this book, but just like the first one, it works well for both extended road trips or while driving on your way to work or to school to pick up the kids.

Combine four ounces of clean water with a dozen drops of peppermint essential oil and tea tree essential oil each. Add each of these ingredients into a spray bottle and shake very thoroughly together, in addition to giving it an extra shake each time before use. This mist is recommended to spray the air inside your car. Avoid getting any of the solution directly into your eyes, ears, or other sensitive areas.

14 – Citronella Lamp Diffusion

This recipe consists of you creating wax cubes (scented ones) to be used in your aromatherapy lamp. This is an alternative to another method where you would add water to the bowl, but this method lasts longer because the wax will not evaporate. You can also recharge it with other essential oils whenever you want.

Combine a half pound of beeswax granules with four ounces of butter, and two dozen drops each of citronella essential oil, geranium essential oil, and cedar wood essential oil.

This recipe is going to require you to acquire some addition equipment, however. You'll need a large pan or bowl in order to simmer water together, a candle lamp diffuser, an ice cube tray (made out of either plastic or silicone), and a large measuring cup made out of glass.

Start by placing the butter and the beeswax into the measuring cup, and then place the cub in the simmering water until the two ingredients have completely melted.

Remove the cup with the butter and beeswax from the water and then allow it to cool for at least fifteen minutes before stirring in the essential oils. Once all of the ingredients have become safely merged together, proceed to pour them into the ice cube tray and put it into your freezer until they become solid.

Once the tray has completely frozen over, pop the resulting wax cubes out of the tray and then place into a zip bag for you to store inside the freezer. You can remove the cubes individually and then place them into your lamp bowl when you see fit. The wax cubes will melt when the candle is lit underneath, and the resulting aroma will fill your room.

15 – Spring Room Spray

Many professional aromatherapists have spoken highly in favor of using lemongrass to calm down the mind and to re-energize it for the next day. This goes perfectly hand-in-hand with springtime.

For your ingredients list, take four drops of lemongrass, two drops each of lemon essential oil and citronella essential oil, and then mix it in with two ounces of distilled water.

The oils should be mixed with some clean water and then poured into a bottle. The delightful scent will refresh everything from your largest family rooms to your smallest closets, so matter where you go in your home; you'll always feel much less stressed.

16 – Basic Eucalyptus Spray Cleaner

This is a safe spray cleaner that makes use of the fresh aroma of eucalyptus to give your home the freshening up it needs.

You'll need approximately thirty two ounces of water, a teaspoon of lavender essential oil, a half teaspoon of eucalyptus essential oil, one quarter teaspoon of Castile soap, and one half teaspoon sodium borate powder.

Mix all of the ingredients together in a spray bottle, and then shake until it has been well blended together. Spray directly onto the dirty surface and then wipe it clean with a cloth or towel. This purifying mixture will get rid of any residue that builds up.

17 – Deodorizing Room Freshener

This mixture will serve well in a container that sits in your kitchen and can be pulled out whenever needed. Combine warm water and a cup of baking soda with two tablespoons of lemon tea tree essential oil.

Stir the ingredients well together until a paste begins to form. Allow this paste to then dry in a flexible cube tray for at least forty eight hours before popping them out and placing one of the molds into a disposer. The remaining molds can then be stored in a jar safely away from children.

18 – Air Freshening Spray

This is one of the freshest and most natural room sprays that you could ask for. The ingredients include ten drops of pine essential oils and fir needle essential oils each, along with three additional drops of tangerine essential oil and four ounces of water.

The oils and water will need to be mixed together in a spray bottle, which you can then proceed to shake very vigorously and then mist any of the rooms in your home.

19 – Winter Diffusion

This is a very straightforward diffusion that will create a very comforting atmosphere in your home during the winter season. Simply take six drops each of orange, clove, and cinnamon essential oils and mix them well together in three tablespoons worth of water. Pour the resulting mixture into a diffuser, and then light a candle to diffuse the mix over the next thirty minutes.

20 – Car Seat Powder

This is an easy to make recipe that should easily be one of your first choices for wiping down the seats in your car. Take a one half cup of baking soda and corn starch each and then mix it with twenty five drops of the first response essential solutions blend.

All of these ingredients will form a powder that's slightly damp when mixed, which can then be very nicely sprinkled over your car seats for a few hours before being vacuumed. If you have any serious stains on any of your car seats, take a bristle brush to make sure the powder gets deep into the stains. Afterwards, you should not only have a very clean car, but a very refreshing one as well.

21 – General Purpose Car Cleaning Wipes

This is a very natural but also creative solution to wiping down nearly any part of your vehicle, from the tires to the dash. The wipes will leave a very clean and citrusy smelling aroma thanks to the pep talk essential solutions oils blend.

For ingredients, merge two dozen ounces of clean water with eight ounces of white vinegar, fifty drops of the pep talk essential solutions oil blend, and a tablespoon of liquid castile soap.

Combine all of the ingredients into your thirty two ounce spray bottle. Use a clean cloth or a paper towel to wipe down the surface when the mixture has been sprayed. The aroma from the mixture will also leave you with a very energizing and invigorating feeling.

22 – Laundry Soap Powder (Lemon and Lavender)

It's easy to see why someone would want to skip over this recipe. There are so many additives and fragrances that have been added to laundry detergent products on the marketplace that it would seem like there's little reason to believe that this recipe would work any better.

However, many of the laundry detergents on the market haven't exactly improved upon one another, and almost all of them are store bought products. This is a recipe that you can make on your own at home with your own resources.

For ingredients, you'll need two cups of sodium carbonate, one bar of Castile soap, two cups of sodium borate, three teaspoons of lavender tea tree essential oil, and then one teaspoon of lemon essential oil.

Use a box grater or a similar device to shred up the Castile soap. Mix all of the ingredients together in a bowl until you come to a damp powder. For each load of laundry (assuming it's an average load), use a quarter cup of the mixture. The leftovers can be stored in a glass container (we recommend that you avoid plastic if you can).

23 – Floors and Furniture Oil

Few people know it, but essential oils mixed with jojoba oil create a very natural yet powerful solution for cleaning up your dusty floors and furniture. The essential oils will do their apart to wipe away the excess grime, while the jojoba oil will be what gives a very nourishing looking and also shielding shine to your floors and furniture.

Combine four ounces worth of jojoba oil with a dozen drops of lemon essential oil, eight drops of sandalwood essential oil, and four drops of lemongrass essential oil.

Mix the essential oils and the jojoba oil into a spray bottle and then shake. Apply small amounts of the mixture to wood floors or furniture, and then wipe it down with a dusting cloth.

24 – Exterior Oven Cleaner

This recipe is similar in function to the previous oven cleaner recipe that we examined, but is instead about cleaning the exterior about your oven rather than the inside.

As a result, the ingredients list is slightly different: one teaspoon of lemon essential oil with a cup of baking soda and liquid soap (preferably unscented) each.

The ingredients can be all mixed together into a bowl until they form a wet paste. Use a cloth, sponge, or a towel rather than a brush to wipe down the outside of your oven with the solution. Keep the oven door closed and the oven off for the duration of the cleaning.

25 – Foot Bath

Several of the body's sensitive nerves and blood vessels that are able to absorb essential oils are found on the feet. But these nerves and vessels will not only absorb these essential oils in the feet, they will also send them throughout the body in order to reduce stress.

There are quite a few more ingredients for this recipe than in previous ones: two tablespoons of salt, one tablespoon of baking soda and white clay powder each, eight drops of lavender oil, four drops of cedar wood and rose oil each, two gallons of hot, clean water, and then one tablespoon each of lavender flowers and rose petals.

First, combine each of the dry ingredients together but leave out all of the wet ones. Then, you can add the essential oils and mix them in evenly with the existing ingredients. The mixture can then be dissolved in a basin that contains over two gallons of warm water. Soak your feet in the basin for as long as you see fit. You'll feel a very balancing and stress-releasing sensation overtaking your body.

26 – Cooling Scalp Remedy

This recipe is designed to both cool and soothe warm heads. Combine six drops of peppermint essential oils, four drops of rosemary essential oils, and an ounce of argan oil into a bottle.

The mixture will then need to be applied directly to your finger tips before transitioning it over to your scalp. We recommend that you shampoo, rinse, and dry your hair before applying this mixture. After you have added the mixture, leave it on for a few minutes before rinsing and styling your hair as you normally would.

27 – Facial Massage

There are a lot of facial creams out there, but many of them are expensive. Here's a facial cream that you can make with your own resources at home and that is more balancing and nourishing than nearly any other kind of normal facial cream products.

All you need is one teaspoon of argan oil, one drop of vitamin E oil, and then three drops of geranium oil. Mix them together and then use your fingertips to dot the mix into your skin's surface and gently massage. Like we said, the resulting balancing sensation you feel on your face will be something that you haven't felt before from other facial cleaning products you've encountered.

28 – Whipped Body Butter

This delightful mixture combine citrus oils with cocoa butter in order to form together a whipped body butter that is among the most moisturizing and aromatic recipes in this entire book.

You'll need four ounces worth of cocoa butter, three quarters cup of coconut oil, one and a half teaspoons of argan oil, and then a teaspoon each of Vitamin E oil and sweet orange essential oil.

You'll also need some additional supplies for this recipe: a mixer, spatula, mixing bowl, two pots, and pint jars.

Use your two pots as a double boiler in order to melt the cocoa butter with coconut oil. Add the argan oil once the mixture has begun to melt accordingly.

Once the mixture has turned into a liquid form, you can then remove it from the heat and add the Vitamin E oil. The oils should start to slightly solidify together again before you can whip them together.

Then, pour the whip into a bowl and mix it for between five to ten minutes. While mixing, add the sweet orange essential oils. Use your spatula to help pour it into jars; with the amounts of the ingredients we've given you, you should have enough to fill up roughly five jars. Cover the jar with an airtight lid.

29 – Scalp Massage

This recipe uses cedar wood and rosemary essential oils to deliver you a very balancing massage for your scalp. Take two drops of cedar wood essential oils and one drop of rosemary essential oil mixed with a teaspoon of olive oil.

Place the olive oil in the palm of your hand first, and then add the essential oils as you rub your palms together. Gently, massage this mix into your scalp, and then use a brush to make sure that it is evenly dispersed around your hair.

30 – Skin Brightener (Lemon)

Lemon essential oil contains a number of properties that come in hand for taking care of your skin. Use three drops of lemon essential oil and lavender essential oil each, mixed with three tablespoons of clean water. After the mixture is complete, use a cotton ball in order to the massage the recipe onto your skin. Avoid any sensitive areas such as your eyes and ear drums.

31 – Mojito Body Scrub

This is a body scrub recipe that will take extra good care of your skin, and is a perfect way to self-treat yourself.

For ingredients, you'll need a tablespoon of jojoba oil and grape seed oil each, three tablespoons of sugar, four drops of peppermint essential oil, and then eight drops of lime essential oil. The oils and the sugar will then need to be mixed together in a small bowl. You can then apply the mixture in circular motions in the bath or shower, and rinse it off thoroughly afterwards.

If you decide to store large amounts of the Mojito Body Scrub for later use, store it in a glass container (avoid plastic) and keep it in a cool and dimmed or dark location. Rooms where the sun shines through the windows all day are not ideal locations for storing this recipe.

32 – Nurturing Facial Cream

This is a delicate cream that makes use of the geranium essential oil (which has a scent very similar to a rose) and doubly serves as a makeup remover.

The ingredients of this recipe consist of a half ounces of beeswax, thirty drops of geranium, carrot seed oil, and lavender essential oil, along with three ounces of clean water and jojoba oil each.

Melt the jojoba and the beeswax in a double boiler (which can be accomplished by having two pans) until the wax fully melts. Remove this mixture from the heat and cool it until it becomes lukewarm before adding essential oils. Warm the water and then pour it into a blender.

Turn on the blender and then add the essential oils/wax mixture in a slow stream. Blend until a cream begins to form, at which point you can store it in a jar to be kept in your refrigerator until needed.

33 – Alternative Nurturing Facial Cream

This recipe is an alternative to the recipe that we just went over. Like that recipe, this one makes use of a rosy scented geranium essential oil to create a cream that will provide a very balanced and nurturing feel to your face, and like the other recipe, can be also used to remove makeup.

Keep the one half ounces of beeswax, three ounces of clean water, and thirty drops of geranium essential oil and lavender essential oil from the last recipe. However, for this alternative we're going to remove the jojoba oil and replace it with an equal amount of rosehip oil (as the two often do not mix together well).

After this, the directions between the two recipes are incredibly similar. Melt and mix the rosehip seed oil and wax together in a bowl before removing it from the heat and allowing it to cool. Add in the essential oils and warm up the water before placing it in a blender. The mixture will then come together as a cream when it blends, and is then ready to be stored in a refrigerator until desired use.

34 – Sauna Blend

For this recipe, you'll need twenty drops of pine essential oil and lemon essential oil each, along with five drops of wintergreen essential oil and birch essential oil each. Combine all of the essential oils together and then add them to a bowl of boiling water. Inhale the resulting aroma from the bowl to receive a very refreshing feeling.

35 – Perfume Oil

This is an essential oil that contains no synthetics, but still provides a very musky and alluring scent. You'll need ten drops of patchouli essential oil, eight drops of cedar wood essential oil, a dozen drops of vanilla essential oil, and one ounce of grape seed oil next.

Combine each of these ingredients together and then mix them together well. Pour the mix into a bottle and allow it to stand as it is for at least three days before applying it. Remember to shake the mixture before using and only apply a few drops at a time.

36 – Summertime Body Lotion

This is a classic do it yourself (DIY) recipes that is excellent for the summer thanks to its lavender scent.

For ingredients, mix together a cup of sweet almond oil, three quarters of an ounce of beeswax, a cup of warm water, three quarters teaspoon worth of lavender essential oil and lemon essential oil each, and then twenty five drops of grapefruit essential oil.

Start by measuring the beeswax and the almond into a bowl. Then, place the bowl into a larger bowl filled with hot, simmering water and wait until the beeswax has completely melted. This mixture can then cool until it becomes hazy, at which point you can place the liquid into a blender. Blend the mixture until it becomes a cream, and then add in the essential oils and store in a cool jar in your refrigerator.

37 – Purification Recipe

This refreshing recipe can be used to fight against aches in your body and encourage open breathing. You'll need fifteen drops of eucalyptus essential oil and grapefruit essential oil each, followed by eight drops of tea tree essential oil.

Sprinkle up to two tablespoons of the rolled oats into a bath. Step into the bath to soften your skin and relieve any itchiness, aching, or irritation that you feel.

38 – Cologne Mist

Rosemary is used in the world of aromatherapy to fight against fatigue and exhaustion in the nervous system. Rosemary has such as powerful effect on both of these things that it is not recommended for individuals who have high blood pressure levels or who suffer from epilepsy.

For ingredients, you will need eight ounces of clean water, six drops of rosemary essential oil, a dozen drops of lemon essential oil and bergamot essential oil each, and then five drops of lavender essential oil.

Pour this mixture into a spray bottle and then shake it vigorously before each use. Spray the mist over the exposed skin to give yourself an energizing feeling.

39 – Skin Saver

For ingredients, you'll need three drops of rose essential oil along with one drop each of carrot seed essential oil and chamomile essential oil.

Wash your hands and face down thoroughly before applying. Then drop each oil onto the palm of your hands and massage it onto your neck and face, while trying to concentrate on the dry areas of the skin. Dry skin can be an impediment to essential oils, which is why you can be a little more liberal this time as you apply it. Hopefully, the dried skin will be pulled away to expose the fresh skin underneath.

40 – Sunny Day Hair Protector

This conditioning oil can be used on your hair before you go for a swim in the pool or step out under the sun alike. It can also protect your scalp and hair from the outside elements including harmful pool chemicals.

What you'll need is one tablespoon of sesame oil and then at least five drops of either lavender or rosemary (your choice here).

Blend the two oils neatly together and then apply them to your scalp and hair, using only a few of the drops at a time.

41 – Spicy Cologne

This spicy but also natural cologne is based in vodka, but it's the vetiver in this recipe that holds all of the scent together.

For this recipe, you'll need three ounces of clean water, an ounce of vodka, twenty drops of bergamot essential oil, five drops of vetiver essential oils, and fifteen drops of bay essential oil.

Start by adding each of the essential oils to the vodka and then stirring them until they are well mixed. Then, add the resulting mixture to the water to dilute it, and continue to stir as you go along.

This recipe should be stored in a glass bottle, and is safe for up to six weeks. Shake the bottle before use and use roughly a half teaspoon at a time on the skin.

42 – Soothing Coconut Body Oil

Virgin coconut oil on its own is excellent for providing a soothing sensation to the body, and it also greatly enhances the aroma effect of this oil.

For ingredients, you will need four ounces of sweet almond oil and coconut oil each, and then one teaspoon of vanilla essential oil and lemon balm essential oil.

To use this recipe, measure the sweet almond and coconut oils into a large measuring cup that's made out of glass. This cup should be bathed in a pan of hot, simmering water until the oils have become completely melted.

At this point, you can proceed to remove the glass cup from the pan, and then stir in the lemon balm and vanilla for an added effect. The completed mixture should then be poured into a glass bottle with a tight cap, to be ready to be applied to your body when desired.

43 – Soothing Muscle Rub

Pine is commonly used in the world of aromatherapy in saunas, massages, and steam baths to help heal sore muscles. This stands in stark contrast to your only other primary alternative, which is to turn to pharmaceutical options. This recipe will greatly aid in soothing your muscles.

You'll need twenty five drops of pine essential oil, peppermint essential oil, and juniper berry essential oil each before adding five drops of lemon essential oil.

Combine each of the oils together in a concentrated blend. The resulting muscle rub will be great after an intense workout or exercise when the muscles are naturally tight or sore.

We suggest that you always dilute the oils with water before applying them to your skin in order to reduce the chance of developing skin irritation.

44 – Vanilla Almond Foot Scrub

For this foot scrub recipe, you'll need a teaspoon of vanilla essential oils, a cup of granulated sugar, a half cup each of whole almonds and sweet almond oil, and a quarter cup of raw coconut oil.

Start by measuring the sweet almond oils and the coconut essential oils in a measuring cup (preferably one that's made out of glass). Place the cup into a bath of hot water until the coconut melts.

At this point, you can then remove the cup form the hot bath. Measure the almonds in a food processor and then grind them up. The grinded almonds can then be added to the melted oils. At that point, simple add in the sugar and assure that everything is well mixed together. You should keep this recipe stored either in a tin or a glass jar.

When using this recipe on your feet, pour the recipe into a basin and then soak your feet until they become soft. At that point, you can then rinse off your feet, dry them down, and massage them. Any of the remaining soil should be rinsed and/or massaged away before you move on to anything else.

45 – Aftershave Gel

This recipe makes use of a very natural aloe gel and a few other essential oils to give you the most nourishing and soothing aftershave that you've ever experienced.

All you need is a cup of basic aloe vera gel, thirty drops each of chamomile essential oil, lavender essential oil, and patchouli essential oil, and then two tablespoons of tamanu oil.

Combine all of these ingredients together in a bowl and mix it together very well. Then transfer the mixtures to a bottle, and use a one half teaspoon at a time by rubbing it in between the palms of your hand and then smoothing it over the shaved area.

46 – Detox Hair Recipe

This hair recipe will require a one half cup of aloe vera gel and bentonite clay powder each, alone with a quarter cup of apple cider vinegar and five drops of Rosemary essential oil.

Mix all four of these ingredients together in a bowl and then work it into your hair. Place a shower cap over your head to keep the ingredients protected as they sit for the next thirty minutes. You don't want to allow the mixture to dry.

Afterwards, rinse your hair out thoroughly, and shampoo your hair approximately thirty minutes after rinsing.

47 – Non-Toxic Deodorant for Sensitive Skin

Each of the aromatherapy recipes for the body that we've explored so far in this book will work wonders for your body. However, some individuals who have very sensitive skin may encounter difficulty in adjusting to a few of these recipes. This recipe in particular is designed specifically for people who have that kind of sensitive skin, because it uses ingredients that tend to have a lesser negative effect on the body.

The recipe's ingredients this time include six tablespoons of arrowroot powder, two tablespoons of coconut oil and bentonite clay, three tablespoons of butter, and one tablespoon of baking soda. You can then also include up to ten drops of an essential oil of your choice (specifically an essential oil that historically has not had a negative effect on your skin).

Add the butter and the coconut oil into a mixer and then whip it until it had been thoroughly mix. Slowly pour in the essential oil of your choice after turning the mixer down to low.

Using a separate bowel, you can then mix together all of your dried ingredients. While continuing to keep your mixer on low, go on to add a third of your dry ingredients. Mix them until they are fully incorporated together. The result should bits of dough within the bowl.

You can then scoop out the mixture and roll it into a ball before placing it into a sealed glass jar to be stored away from sunlight. A tiny amount can then be applied to both underarms each day to provide daily protection.

48 – Cooling Peppermint Toner

This recipe will yield roughly a cup's worth of toner. For ingredients, you'll need a three fourths cup of filtered water, thirty drops of peppermint essential oil, and then a quarter cup of cider vinegar.

Proceed to add the water and the cider vinegar to a spray bottle. Once these two ingredients have been added and thoroughly shook together, you may then proceed to add the peppermint essential oil. We suggest that you start out with the thirty drops like we recommended in our ingredient list, but you can add more if necessary.

Very lightly mist the resulting mixture of your face once in the morning and once in the evening. Alternatively, you can apply it to a cotton ball and then dab it onto your face as well. Keep the spray bottle with the contents stored in your refrigerator.

49 –Rosemary Shampoo

Essential oils are some of the best things we know about for nourishing and cleaning the scalp and hair follicles. Peppermint and rosemary are two of the best essential oils for this task. Not only will they eliminate the oil on your scalp, they can also improve mental cognition and alertness.

The only primary limitation to this recipe is that you should avoid it if you have high blood pressure levels. If this applies to you, you can use lemon or lavender as substitutes.

For ingredients for this recipe, you'll need a one half cup of soap, one half cup of clean water, two drops of peppermint essential oil, and then sixteen drops of rosemary essential oil.

Place the castile soap inside a container that has a flip top, and then proceed to add in both of the essential oils. Mix these ingredients together before adding the cleaned water and then shaking them thoroughly again.

That's all you need to do! From then on, it's only applying a few squirts into your hair and into your shampoo and then rinsing through it as you normally would.

50 – Keeping Pets Off Of Furniture Spray

As much as we love our pet dogs and cats, it's always a pain when they get themselves on the nice furniture and spread their fur around everywhere. This recipe isn't so much about benefiting you physically, emotionally, or spiritually, but rather about keeping your pets off of the furniture so that they'll look nice. Besides, taking the effort to make your home look nicer will better motivate you to trying the other recipes in this book that help make your home look nicer as well.

For ingredients for this recipe, you'll need one and a half teaspoons of peppermint essential oil, lavender essential oil, and lemon essential oil, along with thirty two ounces of water.

Put the essential oils in a spray bottle, and then fill up the bottle with water and shut the bottle very tightly with the sprayer cap. Shake the bottle very vigorously before using, and then spray it two or three times over your target area, and repeat the process over any furniture that you need to.

51 – True Bliss Recipe

This is an incredibly relaxing recipe that is exactly what the title is: true bliss. This is the perfectly recipe after a particularly emotionally charging day that can be breathed in with a diffuser.

The ingredients for this recipe are twenty drops of lavender essential oil, half dozen drops of coriander essential oil and bergamot essential oil, two drops of patchouli essential oil, and a three fourth cups of sea salt. Add up to two teaspoons of skin care oils as well for extra nourishing benefits.

Add 1 or 2 teaspoons of Aura Cacia skin care oils including jojoba, sweet almond and grape seed for extra skin-nourishing benefits.

52 – Emotional Rescue Body Spray

There's a reason why lavender repeatedly pops up as an ingredient in this book. It is easily one of the most versatile essential oils in the world of aromatherapy. It pairs extremely well with other kinds of essential oils and is incredibly relaxing to the body. That's not to mention that it is very easily absorbed by the body as well.

This recipe consists of twenty drops of bergamot and lavender essential oils each, and then one drop of juniper essential oil. Combine each of these with water and then pour them into a spray bottle, and shake it vigorously before using. Apply only two sprays at a time to your body, neck, and face. Keep your ear canals, eyes, and mouth fully covered/closed when spraying.

53 – Lavender Mineral Bath

Chamomile is just one of the relaxing essential oils that pairs very nicely with lavender. It adds more than enough aroma to produce a very balancing effect from this mineral bath.

The ingredients to this bath consist of a half cup of sea salt, six tablespoons of baking soda, forty drops of tangerine essential oil, and thirty drops each of lavender essential oil and chamomile essential oil.

Blend them together in a bowl, and then dissolve a quarter of a cup into a hot bath. Store the remaining mixture in a sealed jar or glass cup, and keep it in a cool and dark location.

54 – Jasmine Bath Brew

For this recipe, you'll need three tablespoons of baking soda, three tablespoons of sea salt, two tablespoons of granules, ten drops of sweet orange essential oil, five drops each of jasmine essential oil and sandalwood essential oil, and a cup of fresh white rose petals.

Combine each of the ingredients together and then sprinkle the mix with the drops of essential oils. You can then pour in the resulting mix into a tub of hot water. This recipe works great with bubble baths as well.

55 - Bath Salts

This recipe is a very relaxing blend of herbs and sea salts to give you a very relaxing bath that delivers both physically and emotionally.

For ingredients, you'll need a cup of sea salt, one teaspoon each of basil, rosemary, sage, and thyme essential oils, and then one tablespoon each of baking soda and lavender flowers.

Combine each of the ingredients in a glass jar and mix them together well. Use just a half cup for each bath.

56 – Lavender Spa Bath

This recipe will help create a very relaxing and luxurious bath experience with a simple blend consisting of one teaspoon of lavender essential oil, three cups of rolled oats, and a third cup of Epsom salt and sea salt each.

The pulse oats should be thoroughly powdered in a blender before being mixed together with Epsom salts, sea salts, and ground oats. The resulting mixture can then be sprinkled with lavender and then blended well together. Dissolve the resulting mixture in a hot bath to yield the truly relaxing effects.

57 – Lavender and Eucalyptus Mineral Bath

You can try this recipe for a very uplifting and herbal filled bath.

You'll need four tablespoons of sea salt, two tablespoons of baking soda, and then eight drops each of chamomile, tangerine, and lavender essential oils. Mix all of the dry ingredients together first before you add the oils. Add one quarter cup's worth at a time to the bath water.

58 – French Clay Powder Bath

This recipe is essentially an extended version of the previous recipe. This soothing bath is a great treat that you can give yourself on a weekly basis, and is excellent for your body, mind, and spirit.

The ingredients here are a quarter cup of baking soda, a quarter cup of sea salt, a quarter cup of Epsom salt, a quarter cup of French white clay powder, a half teaspoon of lavender essential oil, and another half teaspoon of eucalyptus essential oil.

Mix everything together in a bowl, starting with the salts, clay powder, and baking soda and then adding the essential oils later. Whisk until it is well blended together, and then add a quarter cup's worth at a time to the bath water.

59 – Salt Body Scrub

This one is a very stimulating body scrub that will tone and cleanse your entire body. Take four drops of peppermint essential oil, give tablespoons of sea salt, and a one half teaspoon of almond carrier oil.

Mix all three together and then add enough water to effectively dilute the mixture. Apply this mix to the body in circular movements, but be sure to avoid any of the sensitive areas. Rinse off with water after use.

60 – Sweet Lotion Bar

This is a simple homemade lotion that is combines the excellent aroma of cocoa butter and combines it with lavender and lime essential oils to create a uniquely soothing blend that will leave you feeling very smooth.

The ingredients for this recipe include one half teaspoon of lavender essential oil, patchouli essential oil, and lime essential oil each, one teaspoon of Vitamin E oil, one quarter cup of coconut oil, two tablespoons of castor oil and macadamia oil, and one half cup of beeswax and cocoa butter.

For supplies, you will need measuring spoons, a cupcake pan, two pots, a whisk, and cupcake liners if desired.

Start by lining up the mixes in your cupcake pan with the liners. The liners are not completely necessary, but they do ensure that the clean-up process is kept easier. Using a double boiler, mix the cocoa butter and the beeswax over a medium flame. As the mixture begins to melt, you can then add the coconut, macadamia, and castor oils.

The heated mixture should now be a completely liquid, and you can remove it from the source of heat and add the essential oils.

For a final step, whisk it together for at least twenty seconds in order to disperse the essential oils and then pour it into your cupcake pan to complete your new natural lotion bars.

61 – Energizing Liquid Shower Soap

This is the recipe for you if you want a truly energizing aromatic shower. This is perfect while in the middle of a stressed week at work or after an intense workout.

This recipe requires at least twelve drops of cypress essential oil, eight drops of lavender essential oil, two drops of peppermint essential oil, and four ounces of unscented liquid soap.

Mix the oils and the soap together and then use for whenever you need an energizing boost in the shower.

62 – Massage Blend

This aromatherapy massage blend was influenced by several of the traditional Chinese blends that invoke feelings of clarity through the flow of energy. It combines mild energizing aromas with balancing oils.

The recipes for this oil include thirty drops of patchouli essential oils, lavender essential oils, and bergamot essential oils each, ten drops of clary sage essential oils, and five drops of rosemary essential oils.

Combine all of the oils together and then add three drops to an ounce of vegetable oil if you want to use it as a massage oil.

63 – Gentle Facial Mask

This natural face mask relies on essential oils in order to eliminate excess oil. Cornmeal is one of the ingredients that is able to provide this action by removing dead skin cells.

For ingredients, you'll need ten drops of lavender essential oil, five drops of bergamot essential oil, and three drops of clary sage essential oil, three tablespoons of white cornmeal and raw almond meal each, and then three tablespoons of clean water.

Mix the almond and cornmeal together with the essential oils. Slowly stream in the water until a creamy-like paste starts to form together. Apply it to the skin in gentle, circular motions. Allow it to dry out before rinsing it off with warm water, and then pat the area dry with a towel.

64 – Bergamot Deodorant

This is a one hundred percent homemade deodorant recipe that uses a number of ingredients you probably already have in your kitchen, adding to its overall versatility. This also means that you are free from all of the questionable ingredients that several deodorants contain within them.

For ingredients, you'll need a quarter cup of baking soda, five tablespoons of coconut oil, two tablespoons of cornstarch and arrowroot powder each, and then thirty drops of bergamot essential oil.

Blend each of the ingredients together and then place them neatly in a container. To solidify them, simply place the container into a refrigerator. Make sure that your skin is dry and clean before you apply the deodorant.

65 – Lavender and Geranium Bath and Body Oil

This is a very soothing recipe that features both geranium and lavender essential oils, can be used either as a bath oil or as an after bath body oil. For ingredients, you'll need twenty four drops of lavender and geranium essential oil, four fluid ounces of sweet almond oil, and a four ounce bottle.

Mix everything into a bottle, and then measure the sweet almond oil. Add the lavender and geranium essential oils to the bottle, and the shake (assuming the lid has been fully closed) until you're confident the mix is as blended as it could be.

Add an ounce at a time to your bath water, or massage it into your skin following your bath or shower.

66 – Lavender Body Butter

First rate skin care benefits and a very creamy texturing are the front and center features of this recipe.

For ingredients, you need a quarter cup of cocoa butter, one teaspoon of vegetable glycerin, three tablespoons of sweet almond oil, and fifty drops of lavender essential oil.

Melt the cocoa butter in a pan over a low heat. At your best judgment, remove the pan from the heat and then stir in the almond oils, glycerin, and lavender. Transfer the mix to a bowl and set it in a bath of ice water. As the mixture begins to develop pinto a cream, whip it accordingly.

After the cream has fully formed, you can then scoop it into a tin or a jar. Apply whatever desired amount you want to your skin to make a moisturizing cream that's long lasting and delightful.

67 – Lemongrass Tonic

Lemongrass is highly valued in the aromatherapy world for its ability to both re-energize and calm down your mind. Think of a sensation that relieves tension in your body while inspiring you at the same time. That's what the lemongrass skin tonic recipe is all about.

You'll need six drops of lavender essential oil, four drops of lemongrass essential oil, two drops each of chamomile essential oil and clary sage essential oil, and then two ounces of clean water.

Add each of the drops of essential oils to the clean water, and then pour all of it into a spray bottle. Mist your skin while keeping your mouth shut and your ears covered, if possible. The solution should be kept in a refrigerator, so that it will always be refreshed when you bring it out.

68 – Sauna Blend

Pine is one of the ingredients that is often used in massages for sore muscle sand in saunas. It produces a natural evergreen aroma that is an excellent alternative the pharmaceutical options you have.

The recipe list consists of five drops of wintergreen essential oil and sweet birch essential oil each, ten drops of fir needle essential oil, twenty drops of juniper berry essential oil, and then thirty drops of pine essential and lemon essential oil.

Combine all of the oils together, and then proceed to create your own personal sauna as you add several of the drops to a bowl of boiling water. Use a towel as a makeshift tent over your head, and then inhale the mixture by leaning over the bowl to receive the refreshing aroma.

69 – Hot Oil Hair Conditioner

Using an argan hot oil treatment such as this one is a natural and safe way to condition your hair and scalp so long as you do it occasionally.

The ingredients are very simple: only a dozen drops of rosemary essential oil, along with two tablespoons of argan oil.

All of these oils should be thoroughly blended in a glass container, before setting it in a bowl of hot water to bathe it and warm up the oils. The warmed oil can then be worked into your scalp and the shafts of your hair.

Afterwards, wrap your head up in the hot towel and shampoo and condition your hair a few minutes after as you normally would. The resulting sensation is both purifying for your hair and very relaxing for your mind and spirit as well.

70 – Argan Beard Oil

This fresh beard oil combines argan with olive oil and essential oils in order to provide nourishment and protection for your beard.

The ingredients for this recipe include a half ounces worth of whiskey (completely optional), six drops of vetiver essential oil, four drops of bay essential oil, three drops of cedar wood essential oil, and a half ounce of argan oil and extra virgin olive oil each.

Combine the essential oils and the whiskey in a two ounce glass bottle, and then shake it vigorously in order to disperse the oils throughout the bottle.

Add the olive oils and the argan next and shake the bottle very vigorously again. In order to use, you'll need to take a few drops either to your comb or to your hand's palms and then work the recipe into your beard.

The reason we suggest whiskey as a part of this recipe is because it makes the overall recipe lighter. However, it is not at all required and can be replaced by grape seed oil if you would prefer that alcohol be not included in the recipe.

71 – Nourishing Hair and Scalp Treatment

This is a lightly conditioned oil treatment designed to nourish your hair and scalp. It accomplishes this by balancing the essential oils in order to make the treatment more adaptive to any kind of hair.

The ingredients are simple: one tablespoon of rosehip oil, and six drops of lavender essential oil. Blend the two oils together, and then use your fingertips to massage the oils into your scalp and work along your hair as well. Wrap your head in a towel for at least a half hour before removing, and then shampoo and rinse your hair and scalp as you normally would.

72 – Nourishing Facial Oil Serum

This recipe provides absorbing nourishment to your face by balancing rose oils, geranium, and carrot seeds together for a very gentle scent.

The ingredients are a one half ounce of grape seed oil, one half ounce of rosehip oil, six drops of carrot seed oil, and then six drops of geranium essential oil. Mix each of the ingredients together in a bottle with a dropper cap, and then after cleaning it, dot the serum on your face and then smooth it into your skin by using sweeping motions.

73 – Nurturing Facial Cream

This is a delicate facial cream that is designed to balance the geranium essential oils and rosehip seed oils in order to produce a truly nurturing cream.

The recipe consists of twenty drops of carrot seed oil, twenty five drops of geranium essential oil, one ounce of rosehip oil, one half ounce of beeswax, and three ounces of clean water.

Melt the beeswax and rosehip seed oils together in a double boiler until the wax has become fully melted, and then remove this from the heat so it can cool down to a lukewarm level temperature.

At this point, it is safe to add in the essential oil parts of the ingredients before adding the water again. Place the resulting water mixture into the blender in a slow steam, and then blend until a cream begins to form. At that point, you can store the mixture in a jar in the refrigerator and apply it gently to your face when desired.

74 – The Patchouli Blend

This is a very straightforward recipe that yields a rich, fragrant aroma for your next massage or bath. For ingredients, you'll need ten drops of sandalwood essential oil, and then five drops each of patchouli essential oil and rose essential oil. Mix the oils in with a warm bath until they become fully diluted. You can then step in and enjoy.

75 – Patchouli Essence

This recipe produces a very unique but versatile body note for great personal essence. You'll need ten drops of bergamot essential oil, six drops of patchouli essential oil, and four drops of rose essential oil. Combine each of these oils together, and while the results should be fine as they are, the rich aroma can be enhanced even further with the addition of more essential oils such as lemon or lavender. However, neither of these things is completely necessary. Clove and cinnamon can alternatively be used to make it a bit more a spicy fragrance.

76 – Summertime Skin Mist

It's no secret that the summertime is not exactly a good friend of your skin. Fortunately, here is an essential oil recipe that will protect your skin even in the sunniest of summers. This recipe will also provide a very moist sensation to your skin and keep it cool during those hot months as well.

For ingredients, you'll need a dozen drops of spearmint essential oil and peppermint essential oil, two dozen drops of lavender essential oil, a half teaspoon of sweet almond oil, and four ounces of water.

Combine the sweet almond oil, water, and essential oils together in a spray bottle. Shake the bottle very vigorously and then lightly mist it onto the skin. Store the bottle in a refrigerator an ice chest to cool it down if necessary. The primary benefit of this recipe is that it will be very soothing for your skin when it becomes irritated by the sun and the wind.

77 – Mind Clearing Diffusion

This is a very minty and cool peppermint that will give you a very uplifting feeling in your mind in times of stress. A candle lamp diffuser is required for this recipe in order to create the atmosphere of a peaceful state of mind.

For ingredients for this recipe, you will need a half of a dozen drops of sweet orange essential oil, two drops of patchouli essential oil, four drops of peppermint essential oil, and three tablespoons of water.

Place each of the ingredients with water in the bowl of a candle lamp, and then light the candle. The recipe should diffuse for at least thirty minutes, giving you a half hour of an uplifting and calmed down peace of mind.

78 – Orange Foot Scrub

This is a very cooling foot scrub that features orange essential oils and peppermint in order to help relax and clean your tired feet after a day of heavy walking or exercising.

The ingredients for this recipe are a two thirds cup of granulated sugar, two dozen drops of peppermint essential oils and sweet orange essential oils each, and then one ounce of apricot kernel oil.

Measure the sugar and then place it along with the essential oils into a tin or jar. Take a spoon and stir all of the contents of the jar together until it is well mixed. Scoop out a tablespoon at a time to use and massage it into your feet. When completed, rinse it away with warm water and then dry with a towel before moving on.

79 – Lavender and Rose Facial Cream

Rose oil is commonly used in the world of aromatherapy due to its very calm effects. It's a very comforting and powerful aroma that helps to balance sensitive skin. When applied onto a face that has been freshly washed, this recipe is a very sweet-smelling and soothing fragrant.

For ingredients, you'll need four ounces of jojoba oil, three ounces of clean water, twenty drops of rose essential oil, fifteen drops of lavender oil, and then a half ounce of beeswax.

Melt the wax in with the jojoba oil by using a double boiler (which can be done by using two pans). Then, add the cleaned water carefully while also beating the mix with a whisk. Remove the bowls from the heat and until to whisk the mix while adding each of the new essential oils in the ingredients list by drop.

80 - Wintertime Essential Oil Blend

This recipe consists of an excellent combination of essential oils for use during the winter. It makes use of oils from thins such as fir needles and pines, and has a sweetened effects thanks to the welcome addition of juniper and bergamot.

You'll simply need ten drops of cedar wood essential oils, twenty drops of bergamot essential oil, fir needle essential oil, and sandalwood essential oils each, completed with twenty five drops of juniper berry essential oil.

Combine all of these oils nicely together, and for an added effect to make this a massage oil, dilute a dozen drops of vegetable oil into the blend. To diffuse this mixture into the air, place this blend along with a quarter cup of water into a candle lamp and turn it on. The air will fill with the aroma of the blend and you can breathe it in for a very balancing sensation.

81 – Balance Combination Skin Recipe

This recipe makes use of argan oil in order to enhance your skin care and to balance any stubborn skin. It also makes use of the Ylang Ylang essential oil which is incredibly calming. All in all, this is an excellent recipe to take before going to bed each night as it makes you feel more calm and relaxed before going to sleep.

For this recipe, add the Ylang Ylang and the Argan Oil to a small bowl, and then lightly tip your finger tips into the bowl and massage it onto the skin. For another way, you could use a sponge.

82 – Daily Use Argan Oil Skin Care Treatment

When combined with geranium essential oils, argan is an excellent blend for oil skin care from dry to oily to sensitivity skin. The addition of geranium to this mix makes it a very soothing addition to aromatherapy, and is perfect for early use in the morning. When you're feeling relatively low on energy in the morning and need a boost, this is the recipe for you.

Take a small amount of the geranium and argan oil to a jar and gently stir the two together. Massage it into your skin using either a sponge or your fingers.

83 – Wrinkle Reducing Recipe

Many of us, if not all of actually, simply dread the onset of wrinkles. It's therefore perfectly understandable for why you would want to seek out any kind of a treatment that you can find for reducing the onset of wrinkles as much as possible. It would also make sense that you would hope for that solution to be as natural and as relaxing as possible.

Fortunately, you can have it both ways with our wrinkle reducing recipe. This aromatherapy treatment is also very useful for reducing acne in addition to wrinkles as well.

The primary ingredient of this recipe is rose essential oil, which is very soothing, uplifting and motivating for your mood. So whenever you're feeling down and/or want to get rid of any wrinkles or acne that are developing on you, this is the recipe that should be on the top of your list.

Simple take the five drops of the rose essential along with five drops of argan essential oil and then dilute them in with water in a small bowl. Use your finger tips to collect a few drops and then massage them directly into your skin.

84 – Homemade Deodorant Recipe for Extra Sensitive Skin

Yes, that's right; we have yet another deodorant recipe for you here. But then again, there's no reason to be disappointed over it either. If you can find a homemade recipe that works just like another deodorant bar like what you wouldn't find at the store, why wouldn't you at least try it?

The primary benefit for this recipe here is that it is intended for extra sensitive skin. Many people realize the benefits of aromatherapy and try to use essential oils, but are simply unable to because their skin is too sensitive to come into contact with the essential oils. This is a recipe that not only works just as well as the other recipes in this book, but it also works very smoothly with sensitive skin.

The ingredients for this recipe are at least two empty deodorant tubes, ten drops of lavender essential oil, four tablespoons of coconut oil, and a quarter cup of arrowroot powder.

85 – Muscle Soreness Relief Blend

Anyone who has embarked on the road to good health can likely tell you of three different things: eat healthy foods, avoid processed ingredients, cook and grow as much of your own food as you can, and use natural means in order to enhance your body rather than making use of unnatural and fake stimulants.

The muscle soreness relief blend consists of the ingredients of six drops of tea tree essential oil, six drops of peppermint essential oil, six drops of frankincense essential oil, three teaspoons of coconut oil, and three drops of clove.

Mix all of the ingredients together and then massage them into your muscles. Avoid allowing the mix to come into contact with any sensitive areas of your body, such as the mouth, ears, or the eyes, as this mixture is more intense than some of the other recipes in this book. Fortunately, the relief that you feel from this recipe will be great, especially after a good workout.

If you do feel that the recipe is a little too much for you, you can always reduce or even completely eliminate the peppermint essential oil from it.

86 – Immune Booster Recipe

This recipe is intended to give you a boost when you feel bad during the flu and cold seasons. This recipe consists of one drop each of orange essential oil, cinnamon bark essential oil, eucalyptus essential oil, rosemary essential oil, and clove essential oil.

87 – Hair Care Recipe

In this recipe, you can use rhassoul clay and apply it to your scalp and hair. Take a comb and make sure that the mixture is evenly distributed throughout your head and scalp. Rinse it thoroughly with water, then comb again, and then rinse again. We generally recommend against the use of conditioner with this recipe, but if you still strongly desire one, contact a professional aromatherapist. Rhassoul clay is used in this recipe because it is commonly used for deep conditioning in the hair and scalp.

This recipe consists of a one half cup each of rhassoul clay and coconut milk, a quarter cup of herbal water and clean water each, and then one tablespoon of extra virgin olive oil (coconut oil can serve as an alternative if need be).

Start by mixing all of the ingredients together except the oil. Once the mix starts to come together as a paste, you can then add in the oil and stir it accordingly. We suggest that you add just a hint of honey in there in order to enhance the overall conditioning treatment.

Apply the mixture to your hair and allow it to sit with a moist towel wrapped around your head for at least an hour. Afterwards, you can then rinse and style your hair as you normally would.

88 – Grapeseed Lip Balm

This recipe is the only recipe in this entire book that does not have much of a scent, namely because grape seed does not have much of a scent.

The ingredients for this recipe are one tablespoon of grape seed oil, and then one teaspoon each of butter and beeswax.

Combine all three into a double boiler. Once the beeswax has melted, re-pour the mixture into a pot. This is a very fun and easy recipe to make, but like we said, just don't expect it to have the same level of aromas as some of the other recipes in this book. Later on, we'll introduce you to a peppermint lip balm, which is a considerable step up from this recipe. If you're intimidated at the thought of immediately jumping into the peppermint lip balm, however, this recipe is a great way to lead you up to it.

89 – Herbal Infused Lip Balm

For this recipe, you'll need two tablespoons of almond oil, one tablespoon of coconut oil, fifteen drops of peppermint essential oil, and then one and one third tablespoons of beeswax.

Use a double boiler to melt the coconut oil and the beeswax together. Next, add in the almond oil and stir it with a stick or skewer. Once everything has melted well together, you can then stir in the essential oils. Just remember that this will start up fast so you'll need to pour the mixture into your glass jars and containers very quickly before it hardens.

90 – Peppermint Lip Balm

You might be surprised to see peppermint lip balm in this book since it sounds like a more daunting recipe than many of the other ones we have up here. On the contrary, it's one of the easier ones. Plus, if you are able to make a stick of it at a time, that stick will be around for at least the next week.

Obviously there are a few other essential oils that you could supplement for peppermint in this recipe, but peppermint is still our preference and therefore also our suggestion.

For ingredients for this recipe, you will need a tablespoon of beeswax, coconut oil, beef tallow, and butter each, and an empty tube of lip balm, and then at least two drops of peppermint essential oil (though again, there are other essential oils that you can supplement in peppermint's stead if desired, provided that they are safe.

The directions are even simpler than the ingredients. Simple mix all of the ingredients together well and then heat them, pour them into the lip balm tube, and then allow it to cool. You will then have a tube of natural lip balm that should last you for at least a week.

91 – Natural Dandruff Free Shampoo

Dandruff is caused by a number of different things, including but not limited to dry skin, not getting enough shampoo, or extremely sensitivity to normal hair care products.

If the reason that you have been getting more dandruff is because you are sensitivity to the hair care products, than the best cure would be to change to a natural shampoo or conditioner. This will also be a solution for you if the issue is not getting enough shampoo.

The best kind of natural dandruff free shampoo is a lemon essential oil and coconut essential oil combo. Mix two tablespoons of each and then apply it directly to your scalp. Try to avoid letting it coming into contact with your eyes if at all possible.

Allow it to sit for at least five minutes and then rinse it out, but avoid using shampoo if you have long hair. If you have short hair you'll encounter no problems, but with long hair you won't exactly be making the greatest fashion statement in the world, as in your hair could look very clumpy.

If you do have long hair, allow the lemon-coconut mixture to sit for at least an hour before you go back out in public, and then shampoo it out after that.

Coconut oil has been used as moisturizer in many countries for hundreds of years, but even so, not all people react to it well. If you develop any form of an allergic reaction with the coconut oil after applying it, you should absolutely quit taking it.

92 – Raw Honey Shampoo

For the raw honey shampoo recipe, you'll need one tablespoon of raw (or unpasteurized) honey, along with three tablespoons of filtered, clean water and three drops of carrot seed essential oil. When making this shampoo, you'll want to make it on a single service basis to avoid it going spoiled. This is why we're only including a small amount in this recipe.

Heat the mixture slightly over low heat so that the honey can better dissolve. Next, add your three drops of clean carrot seed oil. The oil will add a fragrance to the mixture and also help to get rid of any flaky issues in your scalp, and is very nourishing.

Next, wet your hair and then massage the honey shampoo into your scalp. Make sure that the mix becomes well distributed over your head, and try to focus on actually getting it into your scalp instead of just into your hair. You'll want to rinse it out with water afterward, but there's no need to follow up with any kind conditioner.

93 – Aluminum Free Deodorant Stick

Believe it or not, but you can actually make your very own aluminum free deodorant stick. The ingredients for this recipe should be enough for at least three regular sized deodorant sticks. If that's more than what you believe you need, you can easily cut this down to only half of the recipe that we'll tell you:

You'll need two tablespoons of beeswax, one tablespoon of butter, five tablespoons of coconut oil, a quarter cup of cornstarch, another quarter cu of aluminum free baking soda, a dozen drops of lavender essential oil and tea tree essential oils each, and then at least two or three empty but clean deodorant tubes.

94 – Tallow Balm

This one is a more popular do it yourself item even outside the world of aromatherapy. It consists of three tablespoons of tallow, two teaspoon of extra virgin olive oil, and then eight drops of lavender essential oil.

Mix all of the ingredients together in a stick blender after heating them, and then pour the resulting solution into a glass container. Allow it to cool down and then enjoy.

The reason why we recommend tallow balm is because it's great for repairing scars, for getting rid of acne, and also for moisturizing your skin which is always good for your body. You could even be able to include this recipe as a part of your daily routine.

Another advantage to using tallow balm is that it holds up very well for multiple months when stored in cool and dark locations such as the cupboard. The smell of the tallow balm is also kept to a minimum and will be overlooked by the aroma produced by other essential oils, such as the lavender in this recipe.

95 – Lavender Body Scrub

For this recipe, you'll need two cups of Epsom salt, one cup of organic extra virgin coconut oil, one teaspoon of cut rosemary leaves, and twenty five drops of lavender essential oil.

Take a large bowl, and then add the Epsom salt, rosemary leaves, and lavender essential oil. Mix all of these ingredients together very well, before transferring them to a glass cup or jar.

96 – Homemade Deodorant

It's always better when you can make your own personal hygiene products at home instead of having to buy the products from the store, right? This homemade deodorant recipe will be perfect for this.

All that you need are six teaspoons of coconut oil, a quarter cup of aluminum free baking soda, another quarter cup of arrow root powder, and then fifteen drops of lemon essential oil.

Combine the arrowroot powder and the baking soda together in a bowl, and then mix it thoroughly together with a fork. Proceed to mash the coconut oil in until you start to see a nice paste. At that point, simply add in the essential oils and it's ready to be scooped neatly into a jar. You can then use it as needed. The smell on its is very refreshing and will work wonders for your soul and mind.

97 – Non Toxic Bubbles

This recipe will make about six ounces of non toxic bubbles that you can add to your next bath. All you will need is a half cup of clean water, a quarter cup of dish soap (preferably unscented), and fifteen drops of any kind of essential oil of your choice as long as it is kid friendly, and then one tablespoon of glycerin. Mix all of these things together into your next bath and you should be all set for a very calm and balancing experience.

98 – Coconut Oil Sunscreen

Many people are not aware of this fact, but coconut oil is actually a sunscreen. It may be hard to think about it, but when you are getting ready for a day and a sun and need some UV protection, coconut oil is really all you need.

To prove this to you, Pacific Islanders have been utilizing coconut oil as a sunscreen for thousands of years. It only naturally begs the question for why we would continue using sunscreen products that contain toxic chemicals in them when you could just as easily use a completely natural substance instead.

Some people avoid using coconut oil as a sunscreen, despite its rich history of being used as one, because they believe it could crisp their skin. In reality, if you use coconut oil regularly you should probably never encounter another sunburn for some time.

Just remember to re-apply coconut oil more often, as it only blocks about twenty percent of the total UV rays. You'll also want to use coconut oil in conjunction with not staying out in the sun all day to solidify the high chance of you never getting another sunburn.

Just remember, you always need to at least some sun to hit you, since it's good for you health by increasing your Vitamin D levels. For this reason, you never want to block out one hundred percent of the sun's rays.

It's certainly sad to think about it, but a lot of the sunscreen products currently available on the shelves contain ingredients that are both toxic and can even cause cancer. Anything that comes into contact with your skin can become absorbed by your body, and many of the toxic chemicals that can initiate cancer have a very high absorption rate. This is why you will want to be very wary of sunscreens that claim to be all natural on their labels.

The safest and most effective options, therefore, are to use natural methods such as coconut oil. All that you literally need is just a simple jar of coconut oil like the one in your kitchen. When it's in its hardened form, you can scoop out a few tablespoons worth of it and then apply it directly to your skin. It will rub on to your body just like an ordinary cream.

As an alternative to this method, you can also use coconut oil in liquid form (meaning it's likely been melted), and you can then pour it into a squirt bottle to apply directly to your skin.

99 – Sugar Body Scrub

This recipe is completely homemade, able to be made on a very limited budget using some items that you probably already have in your house, and is very nourishing to your skin.

The recipe is extremely simple, and like we just said, you should already own many of these items: a teaspoon of cinnamon, a cup of packed brown sugar, a teaspoon of Vitamin E, and a half cup of coconut oil.

Start by combining the cinnamon and the brown sugar together in a bowl. Then, add the Vitamin E and coconut oil and mesh it well together with a spoon. The mixture should then be stored in an air right container.

100 – Homemade Body Wash

As the title of our second to last recipe suggests, this is a general purpose body wash that you can make on your own at home. All you need are five drops of lavender essential oil, three teaspoons of Vitamin E oil, two teaspoons of vegetable glycerin, a two thirds cup of castile soap, and then a one half cup of coconut milk.

The ingredients should all be combined in a bottle, and then shaken vigorously before each use. Remember to apply it using either a clean washcloth or sponge.

Tips for Using Essential Oils

There is a lot of information about essential oils out on the web and in other resources. Many resources teach you why you should use essential oils and which specific essential oils you should use, but not nearly as many resources out there tell you about how to actually use the essential oils as well.

The purpose of this chapter is to give you some of these tips on essential oils that are more difficult to find in other resources. Safety in using essential oils should be one of your top priorities when utilizing aromatherapy.

1. All of your essential oils should be stored in a cool and dark location. The purpose of this is to make sure that their quality is preserved for as long as possible. Examples of where you can store your essential oils include in a case within a dresser drawer, or in their very own storage boxes. Either way, essential oils should still

be kept away from electronic outlets so that the frequencies don't disturb the oils.

2. Contrary to what some people may say, you should still feel absolutely free to layer an essential oil on top of another one. Nonetheless, you still won't want to layer more than two blends together. If you do, you run the large risk of mixing the essential oils inappropriately and change up their chemical properties. That's why we recommend that you only blend two or more essential oils that you know are fine when mixed together, but largely avoid mixing two or more blends together, unless of course if your professional aromatherapist gives you permission.

3. Understand the differences between neat essential oils and diluted essential oils. Neat essential oils are oils that have been undiluted, while essential oils that have been mixed in with carrier oil are referred to as diluted oils. Carrier oils are oils that are blended with essential oils when applied to the skin in order to allow the skin to better absorb and spread out the essential oils. Examples of carrier oils include coconut, apricot, olive, sesame, and sweet almond oil.

4. When using citrus essential oils, you need to be aware about the link that exists between them and the sun. Most prominently, you want to avoid applying citrus essential oils to skin that you will be exposing to the sun within the next two days. This is because citrus essential oils are photosensitizing. In simpler terms, they enhance the sun's rays that can cause your skin to either darken or rash. Examples of citrus essential oils include oranges, lime, lemons, mandarin, grapefruit, and tangerine.

5. Never apply more than five drops of essential oils at a time. In fact, five drops on its own is far too much! Most experts recommend only one to three drops at a time.

6. Most experts also recommend that you dilute your essential oils as much as possible. The reason why you would want to dilute them is because they can then spread out over a larger area and absorb into the skin faster. The more time your oils spend on your skin when they are absorb better, the more effective they will be. However, the level to which you dilute your essential oils should depend on how sensitive your skin is.

7. If you do have sensitive skin, you should avoid hot essential oils if at all possible. Hot essential oils are oils that produce a burning or warming sensation when they come into contact with the skin. This causes obvious problems in people who do have sensitive skin, especially young children and infants. Examples of hot essential oils include lemon, peppermint, cinnamon, clove, oregano, basil, thyme, and black pepper. Remember that one of your top goals when using aromatherapy is safety, and that means if your skin is sensitive, you need to avoid the oils that will make your skin worse.

8. Speaking of essential oil safety, always keep any kind of essential oils away from your eyes as much as possible. Just to be on the safe side, you'll want to avoid letting the oils come into contact around your eyebrows and the cheekbones. You also need to be careful that you don't rub your eyes after using the essential oils without washing or rinsing your hands. In the event that you do get some essential oils, never use water to try to wash away the pain. Instead, use a drop of olive oil. It really does help. Even though it sounds weird, it won't deliver any pain to your eyes. The reason why you should use olive oil instead of water to stop any other essential oils that have gotten into your eyes is because water will only spread out the oils, while olive oil will drop it out.

9. If there are any directions in using any kind of an essential oil, always follow them! This means read up on the labels and conduct any research on that particular oil that you can. The labels will tell you the ingredients of the

oils (so you can avoid any kind of an allergic reaction), as well as how they can be taken, such as through inhalation or in direct contact with the skin.

10.   Remember to follow some specific safety procedures when using the essential oils in the respective way that they can be taken. When inhaling essential oils in aromatherapy for instance, you should always diffuse with a diffuser, or place a few drops in your hand's palm and then breathe it in deeply. When allowing the oils to come into direct contact with your skin, drop the oil right into your skin and then rub it carefully together. When swallowing an essential oil, always place them into clear vegetable capsules and then swallow them down with water.

11. Avoid using plastic bottles when conducting aromatherapy and still to glass bottles, especially if you're adding essential oils to water. The reason for this is because the majority of essential oils have chemical properties that allow them to break down both Styrofoam and plastic. This means that you would essentially be consuming or coming into contact with both the essential oils and the plastic, which you want to avoid.

12. Talk to other people who use aromatherapy and seek their input. It is extremely helpful when you hear about another individual's positive experiences with aromatherapy, or hearing about mistakes they made that you can avoid. If you don't personally know anyone who does do aromatherapy, look or testimonials online. You can also attend classes if available in your local area.

13. While not necessarily a true safety tip, it's still important to know how much oil is in each bottle you buy. Most fifteen milliliter bottles will contain roughly two hundred and fifty drops worth of essential oils. For bottles that have a volume of roughly five milliliters, the number of drops is closer to one hundred.

14. Examples of oils that contain just one kind of oil include peppermint, lavender, oregano, grapefruit, lemon, thyme, and so on. This differs from the term 'blend' that is used in the world of aromatherapy and is used to refer to a formulated combination of these kinds of oils.

15. Just like how you want to keep essential oils as far away from your eyes as possible, you also want to keep them as far away from your ears and ear canals. Never place essential oils in your ear canal. While it is okay to rub them around your ears, especially around the pressure points behind the ear or on the lobe, you must be very careful to never actually place a drop of oil in your ear at all.

16. Knowing about dilution ratios is important in aromatherapy. When an essential oil is 'neat' it means that it has been completely undiluted. When the term 'fifty-fifty' is used, sometimes written as 50:50, it means that exactly one essential oil has been diluted with exactly one pet carrier oil. When the term 'twenty-eighty' or 20:80 is used, it means that one essential oil has been diluted with four carrier oils. Most professionals recommend that you dilute your oils to at least one degree.

17. Most professionals in aromatherapy recommend that you test out an essential oil before using it constantly. Take at least two or three drops of carrier oils and mixing it in with essential oils, before rubbing it into a small part of your skin. If you feel any sensitivity in your skin, it means either that you need to dilute the oils even more OR weight at least two or three weeks until your body is able to become accustomed to the new benefits of the oils.

18. It's best that you avoid using essential oils with children who are under eighteen months, but you especially don't want to let essential oils come into contact with the neck or throat of these young children. While rare, there are a few specific kinds of essential oils that

you will want to avoid using with children under the age of twelve. Do your research.

19. Speaking of children, your essential oil bottles should be kept out of a child's reach in general. Treat your oils as you would any other kind of medication and teach your kids that they are not allowed to touch the bottles.

20. Finally, always conduct more research on aromatherapy and seek to always expand your knowledge in the field. While this book has done much to teach you what aromatherapy is, the health benefits of it, and over a hundred of the different kinds of recipes that you can use, you can never learn too much. Look for more resources where you can learn the safest and most efficient ways to use essential oils in aromatherapy.

Conclusion

In this book, we have learned what the basic principles of aromatherapy are and the numerous health benefits that they can give your body and mind. We then examined one hundred and one of some of the most effective aromatherapy recipes out there, using a variety of oils and different ways that they can be taken. Finally, we provided you with twenty safety tips on using essential oils.

If you want to establish a firm connection between your mind, body, and spirit, then aromatherapy is the treatment for you. Try just a couple of the recipes we have provided you with and witness the wonders that they can provide.

Thank You For Reading!

If you enjoyed this e-book, then please share your thoughts by leaving a review on Amazon!